Parathyroid Glands

A Patients Guide

Andrew McLaren FRCS
Consultant Surgeon

Table of Contents

Primary Hyperparathyroidism – or how they go wrong

The parathyroid glands are tiny and live in the neck.

Most people have 4 glands and they usually sit on the back of the thyroid gland – para meaning 'near to' the thyroid gland.

Parathyroid glands have nothing to do with the thyroid gland and the two different endocrine glands function entirely separately.

What do Parathyroid Glands Do?

The 4 parathyroid glands sit next to the thyroid gland, which is just below your Adams Apple – or voice box.

Each of the parathyroid glands plays a part in controlling the level of CALCIUM in your body and in particular in your blood. The parathyroid glands make a hormone called parathyroid hormone – commonly abbreviated to PTH. It is the parathyroid hormone which controls calcium metabolism.

Calcium is one of the body's salts and is absolutely crucial to the way muscles and nerves function – but more about that later.

Thermostats

The parathyroids are best thought of as a combination of home central heating boiler and thermostat all rolled into one tiny little structure – the size of a grain of rice.

Each one is trying hard to control the level of calcium in the blood within a narrow range. This range is typically between 2.2 mmol/L and 2.55 mmol/L (8.5 – 10.2 mg/dL USA units).

If the calcium level goes up a bit then they sense this and automatically produce less hormone. If the calcium levels fall they produce more PTH to push the level up again.

PTH doesn't last long in the blood – a concept called half-life describes this as approximately 4 minutes. So if the parathyroid glands stop making PTH the level in the blood of PTH will halve in 4 minutes – this is really quick for a hormone - thyroid hormone by way of contrast has a half-life of 7 days.

So if one of the parathyroid glands becomes overactive this is because the gland has usually enlarged but more importantly the extra cells have faulty thermostats that have been reset to a higher level of calcium.

The remaining normal glands do what they are supposed to do when they sense higher calcium levels and switch off.

What does PTH do?

Parathyroid hormone regulates calcium through its effects on your bones, intestines and kidneys. It doesn't do anything else.

Importantly raised PTH levels do not in themselves result in symptoms.

The commonest cause of an elevated PTH level is a low level of vitamin D.

Parathyroid Action on Bones

Your bones contain 98% of the body's calcium. It is the calcium that makes bones strong and without it they would be bendy and weak.

So bones stay strong throughout life because of a constant remodelling process which means that we are always making new bone and destroying old bone. As a result unlike concrete tower blocks which start to crumble as they age bones can stay healthy because of two special types of cells:

Osteoclasts – these cells destroy or clear out old bone

Osteoblasts – these cells build new bone

Both osteoclasts and osteoblasts are active throughout life constantly building and remodelling bone.

Obviously during childhood when bones are growing the balance is in favour of the osteoblasts building new and bigger bones. Even when growth stops at the end of teenage years there is bone strengthening over the next 20 years or so.

Maximum bone strength is reached in the mid to late 30s.

From here on in the osteoclasts win just ever so slightly reducing bone mass steadily. This process is magnified in women when they go through the menopause and who can lose up to 1% of bone mass each year.

This bone loss is often accelerated by parathyroid disease. I would stress here that the acceleration is minimal and does not affect everybody. Ten years after a diagnosis of parathyroid disease and without treatment half of the people diagnosed will have developed osteoporosis

Parathyroid Development

The parathyroid glands develop from the 3rd and 4th branchial pouches which also contribute to the development of the thyroid and thymus glands.

These pouches develop differently in the embryo and this results in their varying positions in the neck.

Parathyroid Anatomy

Humans normally have 4 parathyroid glands. Some have 5 or more (1-2%).

They are normally situated behind the thyroid gland each in a tiny capsule of tissue with some surrounding fat.

Each gland has a small artery and vein.

The majority are within a small area marked by the crossing of the recurrent laryngeal nerve and inferior thyroid artery.

Superior parathyroid glands can drop down low in the neck – usually in a posterior position and occasionally even behind the oesophagus (gullet). The superior gland when enlarged may even drop down into the chest. On rare occasions the superior gland fails to descend in the development stages and can be found high in the neck.

The inferior glands can be more variable in position. Usually around the back of the lower part of the thyroid gland they may in the fatty connective tissue below the thyroid gland or even in the thymus gland itself. Inferior glands can occur within the thyroid.

Normal parathyroid glands are small ovoid structures – a good approximation is the size of a grain of rice. A rough size would be 5 x 3 x 1mm giving a volume of 15 mm^3.

An abnormal parathyroid gland – commonly an adenoma – is usually enlarged but may not be particularly big. A common size for an adenoma is 10 x 20 x 5 mm – this would give a volume of 1000mm^3 so it is easy to understand why that volume of cells lacking proper regulation would cause a problem.

Parathyroid Pathology

Adenomas – these are the cause of the majority of primary parathyroid disease. An adenoma is a benign growth and in parathyroid glands a number of cell types can enlarge – chief cells, oxyphil cells and water clear cells. Adenomas do not have to be large the key issue is that the cells have lost the normal thermostat mechanism. A characteristic feature under the microscope is that a compressed rim of normal parathyroid tissue can be seen around the periphery.

Hyperplasia – this type of enlargement occurs in 10-15% of patients. Crucially it is more likely to affect all the parathyroid glands although rarely are all equally enlarged. For the surgeon it is important to assess all four glands and make a judgement as to which ones to remove – usually the largest 2 or 3.

Carcinoma – parathyroid carcinoma is rare (less than 1% of cases). Cancers are difficult to diagnose preoperatively and are not easy even when assessing pathology after surgery. Fortunately they are virtually all curable by surgery.

Parathyroid Physiology

PTH secretion is controlled by the level of serum calcium through a negative feedback mechanism.

Each parathyroid cell has receptors sitting on its surface called calcium sensing receptors and if these are activated a lot indicating high levels of calcium then the release of PTH is reduced.

The key here is that PTH is PREFORMED and stored in the parathyroid cells in storage granules. There is almost a permanent background production and release of PTH as it only lasts for a very short time (minutes) in the blood stream.

This short life of PTH is described as a short half-life i.e. the time it takes for half of the PTH in the circulation to be removed which is 4 minutes. Some hormones have a long half-life for example the main thyroid hormone (T4) at 6 days.

Diagnosis of Primary Parathyroid Disease

For the sake of simplicity I do not use the term hyperparathyroidism. It is too long a word and is easily confused. In addition, doctors can confuse it with the rare secondary and tertiary conditions which in general are not something that need considering.

Primary parathyroid disease is simple, easy to say and people know what we are all talking about.

The rules of endocrine surgery are simple and there are but three:

1. Confirm the diagnosis
2. Make the patient safe to operate on
3. Do the correct operation

All this sounds simple but with parathyroid disease it can be quite complicated.

Many patients come to clinic thinking they must have parathyroid disease because they have all the symptoms of it – not necessarily true.

The diagnosis is not based on symptoms but on biochemical tests – of blood and sometimes of urine.

The key to diagnosis is a **raised serum calcium level**. This needs to be the so called corrected serum calcium level which is adjusted for the amount of a protein in the blood called albumin.

So a calcium blood test should always display three results:

Calcium

Corrected calcium

Albumin

A normal albumin level is taken as 40 g/l.

If the albumin is below this then you need to add 0.02 mmol/l to the calcium result and if the albumin is above 40 you need to subtract 0.02 mmol/l to the calcium result to get the corrected value.

All biochemistry laboratories have a reference range for blood tests. Calcium is usually between 2.15 and 2.55 for the corrected serum level. It is important to remember that this range covers 95% of the results for the population. As a result 2.5% of results will be below this range and 2.5% of results above the range yet still be normal.

Interpretation of high calcium results therefore needs extreme caution particularly if just outside the normal range.

Making the diagnosis

In the majority of patients this is relatively easy:

Elevated calcium levels

PTH level either normal (inappropriately elevated) or raised

From what we have said earlier about the parathyroid glands it is clear that if the calcium is higher than it should be the parathyroids should switch off and stop making PTH so the level should be low. Thus a normal PTH level with a high calcium is just as abnormal as a high PTH level.

No surgery should be considered unless there are at least 2 elevated calcium levels to confirm the diagnosis.

Supporting tests include:

High urine calcium – hypercalciuria – this is found by undertaking a 24 hour urine collection and measuring the level of calcium excreted through the kidneys

A high urine calcium is found in approximately 75% of patients. Some patients with true parathyroid disease will have normal levels of excretion.

A very low level of calcium in the urine raises suspicions of another disorder – familial hypocalciuric hypercalcaemia.

In practice it appears that patients with high levels of urine calcium tend not to have particularly high levels of calcium in the blood – presumably because the kidneys are doing a good job of excreting it all.

Patients with high levels of urine calcium are at risk of forming kidney stones if the calcium crystallises out.

Serum alkaline phosphatase – this is an enzyme in the bones and goes up if there is bone disease. Bone disease from parathyroid problems is nowadays quite rare so this test is much less useful.

Symptoms of parathyroid disease are due to the high calcium level

This is a very important statement.

Some patients come along with a single mildly elevated calcium level and a whole series of normal ones – yet they have 'symptoms' every single day.

I am always concerned in this situation as the days when calcium is normal should be symptom free – remember symptoms are caused by the calcium being high.

Calcium is a key salt in the human body and is used to generate muscle contraction in all types of muscle. This includes heart muscle and the gut which contains smooth muscle as well as the obvious arm and leg muscles.

Asymptomatic Parathyroid Disease

The big question with parathyroid disease is what to do when there are no symptoms.

Historically since the first parathyroid operation was performed in 1925 by Felix Mandl the disease has changed.

Back then the classic symptoms were:

- Bone pain
- Kidney stones
- Muscle damage
- Neurological / psychiatric problems

These symptoms can still occur but many patients who turn up with an elevated calcium level on blood testing have none.

The reality however is different.

Many patients who are 'symptom free' have subtle manifestations of parathyroid disease with often vague symptoms. The problem is that these have crept up so gradually as calcium levels rise that the patient doesn't recognise them as 'symptoms' more as every day life.

A number of studies have looked at this issue. A detailed questionnaire study developed by Dr Janice Pasieka, Professor of Endocrine Surgery in Calgary, Canada has been used in several studies.

The questionnaire is given to patients both before and after surgery who have as far as they are concerned no symptoms. The questions test various potential symptoms such as muscle aches, energy levels and thirst.

The results consistently show that 'asymptomatic' patients feel better after successful parathyroid surgery.

The parathyroids are still diseased – bone mineral density (bone strength) is observed to decline in up to 50% of patients with parathyroid disease who do not have surgery.

Parathyroid Disease Treatment

Surgery for parathyroid disease is the ONLY way to provide a permanent cure.

A number of endocrinologists still recommend not treating primary parathyroid disease until calcium levels are "high". This is a view becoming less common as parathyroid surgery has improved and a greater realisation of the disabling nature of the symptoms of parathyroid disease.

There are no good non-surgical treatments. A number have however been tried and these include:

Bisphosphonates – these are bone protecting drugs usually given to treat osteoporosis. Unfortunately they do not treat parathyroid disease and are usually not sufficient to prevent bone damage from parathyroid disease either.

I generally recommend bisphosphonates only after successful parathyroid surgery and preferably with monitoring of effect by your local endocrinology consultant or General Practitioner.

Cinacalcet – this oral drug works by convincing the faulty parathyroid cells that there is more calcium in the blood than there is – conning the thermostat as it were – and thereby reducing PTH levels. In technical terms cinacalcet increases the sensitivity of the calcium sensing receptor which is on all parathyroid cells to extracellular calcium.

The drug dosage is adjusted to maintain a lowered level of calcium. Cost is high at between £15 and £60 per day.

Cinacalcet almost always is successful in controlling the high calcium levels. The drug was first introduced to treat secondary parathyroid disease but has been used successfully in patients with parathyroid disease who cant proceed to surgery.

Side effects of cincalcet treatment do occur – common side effects include:

Blurred vision
Chest pain
Dizziness
Headache
Anxiety

Surgery for Parathyroid Disease

Surgery used to be a major operation and entered into as a last resort however fortunately in many areas of the UK and in specialist centres around the world the surgery has improved.

There are two operations available:

Standard parathyroidectomy

Minimal access parathyroid surgery

Surgeons undertaking parathyroid surgery should be in a position to offer both procedures.

Questions to ask your surgeon:

- How many parathyroid operations do you perform each year?

    This should be a good number e.g., 40 plus

- What is your success rate?

    No surgeon cures every patient they operate on

    Should be over 95% cure

- Do you take part in multi-disciplinary team meetings?

    Best practice involves discussing cases with endocrinology and radiology colleagues to obtain the best results

- Are your radiology colleagues and radiographers specialised?

    As you will see below the quality of imaging in radiology is vital to getting good results – just like surgeons should specialise so should the supporting teams.

Minimal Access Parathyroid Surgery

Removal of a single parathyroid gland through a 2cm incision – yes just 2cm – on the side of the neck. This is called minimal access or minimally invasive parathyroid surgery (MIP).

This is a great operation:

- Performed as a daycase procedure
- Tiny incision
- Almost invisible scar
- Minimal pain – if any
- High success rate

However to perform mini parathyroid surgery requires great radiological imaging and a surgeon who undertakes enough parathyroid operations to be confident.

This is because the faulty parathyroid gland must be **identified** by scanning to allow the surgeon to dive down straight onto it through such a tiny incision.

Requirements for mini-access parathyroid surgery:

- Sestamibi scan shows single hotspot
- Ultrasound demonstrates parathyroid adenoma – however see below
- No previous thyroid / parathyroid surgery
- No previous neck radiotherapy
- Thyroid gland of reasonably normal size

The radioactive Sestamibi scan is crucial to undertaking mini-access parathyroid surgery.

When this scan shows a hotspot on the delayed (2-3 hour) images this means that there is just one faulty gland and gives its approximate position.

When the gland lights up on Sestamibi scanning it is likely to be the single offending gland – crucially important as with minimal access surgery the others will not be seen.

The parathyroid ultrasound pictures are very useful. These provide the surgeon with a road map of where the parathyroid gland is and how to get there.

Most parathyroid adenomas are close to the thyroid gland – either behind it or at the lower tip. When seen clearly on ultrasound the surgeon is able to come through the incision and see the thyroid gland clearly then proceed around the thyroid gland to locate the parathyroid adenoma.

Having performed a large number of mini-access parathyroid operations I am happy to undertake MIP surgery
This is why the team approach with a good and interested radiology consultant and radiographers is crucial.

The radiology consultant undertaking the ultrasound needs to know what a faulty parathyroid gland looks like. They also need feedback from the surgeon on what is actually found in the neck – otherwise they never know the true answer!

I do undertake MIP surgery in patients whose Sestamibi scan is positive but in whom the ultrasound scan has not located the adenoma. This is because after 10 years of performing this type of surgery as a consultant with an excellent radiology team I know that adenomas in these cases are likely to be at the back of the neck – a little too deep for ultrasound to penetrate and therefore see.

This knowledge extends MIP surgery to more of my patients which is a good thing.

Traditional parathyroid surgery

All parathyroid surgery used to be undertaken through a large neck incision.

This was because historically parathyroid surgery was done by surgeons more used to removing the thyroid gland and they did this through a large incision.

More importantly these old-fashioned surgeons also cut the underlying strap muscles in the neck. The strap muscles run vertically in the neck and help maintain a normal contour of this visually important area.

There is no need whatsoever to cut these muscles – cutting a muscle is painful afterwards and causes bruising and swelling. They can never be repaired properly as the fibres run vertically.

Modern parathyroid surgery adopts techniques from thyroid surgery but recognises that only a small space is required in most patients and cuts are therefore much smaller – 5 to 6cm.

As a result modern parathyroid surgery is not a "big deal" and just requires a single overnight stay in hospital.

Once the patient is asleep in conjunction with the anaesthetic team we carefully position the head and shoulders so that the neck is extended which makes access to the area around the thyroid gland much easier.

The operation takes between 30 minutes and 2 hours. The precise timing depends on how easy it is to find all 4 parathyroid glands. As indicated earlier they are quite variable in position and also normal ones are very small so can be tricky to identify.

I use an injection of a small volume of methylene blue dye – done after the induction of general anaesthesia – which can helpfully stain faulty parathyroid glands dark blue making them easier to find.

Superficial cervical plexus blocks

Local anaesthetic put alongside the sternomastoid muscle in each side of the neck will numb the front of the neck and the area inside around the thyroid gland.

This new technique is very important for quality parathyroid surgery.

Numbing up the neck before your surgeon operates means that the anaesthetist does not need to give powerful anaesthetic drugs to overcome any pain during the operation.

With long-acting anaesthetics your neck will remain numb for up to 24 hours.

If your surgeon has just cut the skin and parted the muscles inside along the natural tissue planes there is very little to be uncomfortable therafter – as a result most patients with a specialist surgeon and anaesthetic team will not need any painkillers at all after the surgery.

This is a huge advance on the standard 2-3 nights in hospital offered by many hospitals still in the UK.

As a consequence of using all these modern techniques the majority of my patients do not need any painkillers after surgery.

Complications of Parathyroid Surgery

Scar

Bleeding

Infection

Recurrent laryngeal nerve injury

Failure to cure

Hypo - parathyroidism

Complications are fortunately rare after surgery but it is always important that patients understand the risks and that surgeons appreciate these and attempt to minimise them.

Each of the complications will be considered in turn

Scar

All operations swap the problem inside for a scar. In parathyroid surgery this can be as small as 2cm for the true minimal access parathyroid operation – note this is not the mini-radioguided surgery which some centres in the USA offer through a much larger incision.

At the most the scar will be 5 cm in length.

The cut is placed in a skin crease in the front of the neck and most surgeons go to extreme lengths to place the incision as neatly as possible and as centrally as possible. This improves healing and the symmetry reduces the number of people who will notice something.

Scars take about a year to reach their final healing point and along the way often go through a phase of being quite obvious and maybe reddened. This is all normal and most fade slowly to a fine white line.

In occasional patients the scar can become thickened – hypertrophic in medical language – and this may need treatment but happens in less than 1 in 200 patients.

Keloid scarring can occur particularly in patients with African skin types or who have had similar scarring elsewhere. There are tricks to minimise this and your surgeon will speak to you about it if you are at risk.

Following surgery my personal practice is to use dissolving sutures underneath the skin and then seal the skin with medical skin glue which is essentially a non-irritant form of superglue.

The advantage of glue is that the wound is immediately waterproof and bug proof so patients can shower, wash and even go swimming.

After the surgery it is important to keep stretching the neck gently and then when the wound settles to start gently massaging the neck to help the wound settle down.

Massage is crucial as the skin on the neck is generally quite loose and it is important that it is loose for everything to feel normal. After surgery the layers of skin and muscle tend to stick together which can feel uncomfortable or even painful to some patients.

By massaging the scar, moving it around, you will free up the skin from the underlying muscles and everything settles back down properly.

Bleeding

Bleeding is a recognised complication after parathyroid surgery. Indeed after any surgery bleeding and bruising can occur.

When a surgeon talks about bleeding in the neck they usually mean fairly dramatic bleeding that can happen in the first few minutes after an operation or in the first few hours. The risk of such bleeding is under 1%.

Bleeding in the neck can be serious and may even need a further quick operation to clear the blood out as it can cause obstruction to the airway.

It is for this reason that we tend to keep patients who have had full parathyroid surgery in overnight and allow them home the next morning.

Infection

This is very rare but can happen as in any wound. Antibiotics are not generally given for parathyroid surgery.

Recurrent laryngeal nerve injury

The risk of nerve injury is low (approximately 1 in 200 cases).

The recurrent laryngeal nerves run on each side of the neck. The nerves come into the neck from the chest and travel behind the thyroid gland to insert into the larynx.

Inside the larynx the nerves supply all the intrinsic muscles of the larynx (excluding cricothyroid) and some sensation to the mucosa below the vocal cords.

The effects, or morbidity, of recurrent nerve injury can vary from minimal changes in the voice to marked hoarseness and a lack of power in the voice.

The hoarseness makes it difficult to project the voice and it tires easily.

Patients also describe feeling out of breath.

Injury occurs because the parathyroid glands can be in close association with the nerve and an enlarged parathyroid gland may have to be dissected off the delicate nerve which subsequently doesn't function normally. Usually the nerve and the voice recovers within 4 – 6 weeks of surgery.

Permanent voice injury is rare but there are techniques available to improve voice quality if an injury does turn out to be permanent.

Failure to cure

This complication is one that all parathyroid surgeons worry about as it is the most annoying to a patient who has gone through surgery.

Unfortunately it is not always possible to identify the offending parathyroid glands. They are recognised as being the most variable bit of human anatomy and whilst are commonly in close association with the thyroid can drop into funny little corners of the neck and even drop into the chest.

The faulty parathyroid gland can be very small – bear in mind the normal glands are about the size of a grain of rice.

The smallest adenoma I have removed was a 3mm addition to an otherwise normal parathyroid gland.

Parathyroid glands can also hide within the thyroid gland – thus completely impossible to identify during surgery.

The risk of failing to cure varies with the experience of your surgeon but should be less than 5% of first time surgeries.

Hypo-parathyroidism

Old textbooks of medicine and surgery describe a 'bone hunger' occurring after parathyroid surgery resulting in low blood calcium levels and symptoms from this e.g., tingling around the lips and mouth, tingling in fingers and muscle spasms.

I have only seen low blood calcium after parathyroid surgery once in 10 years – in modern practice it is therefore extremely rare!

What is more commonly seen in patients who have been cured is that when the calcium levels fall into the normal range the body 'perceives' this drop to normal as a 'low' level of calcium.

This is not so stupid as for that patient it is indeed much lower than it has been for some time. Generally the symptoms are just of tinglings in finger tips and around the mouth with no muscle spasms.

The tingling can be relieved by taking calcium tablets but I usually just advise patients to be pleased as it means they are cured and ride the symptoms out. The tingling resolves over a few days in most cases although I have seen it in one patient go on for 3 months – and all the time with a normal blood calcium level.

Permanent hypoparathyroidism should be staggeringly rare but can happen in patients undergoing redo surgery.

Failure to Cure Parathyroid Disease

Nearly all patients undergoing parathyroid surgery will be cured (98%).

There are a small number who are not cured first time round. This is always extremely disappointing but cannot be prevented.

So why is parathyroid disease so difficult:

1. The parathyroids are the most variable bit of human anatomy and can be almost anywhere in the neck
2. Parathyroid adenomas may be very small – I have cured one patient with a 3mm adenoma which was little more than a grain of sand – the cells in them however are faulty
3. Parathyroid glands may be embedded within the thyroid gland – thus entirely invisible to the operating surgeon.
4. Parathyroids may drop into the chest
5. The surgeon may simply not find it on that particular day

After unsuccessful surgery the first thing to do is to get back to normal as quickly as possible.

Then a careful reassessment should be undertaken and this should include a thorough review of all blood tests, urine tests and scans to ensure the diagnosis was correct in the first place.

In young patients careful assessment to exclude familial hypocalciuric hypercalcaemia (FHH) should be undertaken and consideration given to genetic tests for MEN (multiple endocrine neoplasia).

Assuming the diagnosis of primary parathyroid disease is confirmed proceed with further imaging which should include:

1. Sestamibi scan

     Always repeated
     Can change after removal of one adenoma / abnormal gland and reveal the location of a previously unidentified problem gland.
     One of the first patients I did not cure had 2 large adenomas in the neck removed at surgery and 2 normal glands were found. Calcium levels remained high and we repeated the Sestamibi scan to find a 5th gland lighting up dramatically in her chest – this was subsequently removed and confirmed as a 3rd adenoma. This is very rare but illustrates the challenges.

2. CT scan

     CT scanning should be done with intravenous contrast to look at the neck (starting at the base of the skull) and the upper chest (at least to level of mid chest).
     Some parathyroid glands can descend into the chest and be shown using this technique equally some glands may not descend fully and show up high in the neck.

3. Selective Venous Sampling

     This test is done by a consultant radiologist in an xray suite. It involves passing a very tiny catheter into a vein either in the arm or leg. The catheter can be seen by the imaging equipment either with markers along its length or by the injection of an xray contrast medium into the catheter.

The consultant has to guide the catheter through the veins up to the head / neck / chest area.

Blood samples are taken at numerous points through the catheter. Each sampling position is marked on a road map of the veins which the radiologist fills in as they go.

The aim is to take a large number of samples a from the neck and upper chest veins on both sides.

Parathyroid hormone level is then measured on all the individual samples. The general principle is that the highest reading indicates the point closest to the offending parathyroid gland.

This test is invasive and time consuming but has a very low complication rate. It is considered extremely useful in difficult cases and in particular for confirming that the offending gland is in the chest before surgery.

Parathyroids and Osteoporosis

Osteoporosis is defined as the loss of bone strength with thinning of the bones measurable on bone density scans (DEXA scans).

Calcium provides the strength to the bones and 98% of all the calcium in the human body is in the bones.

Bones remain strong throughout life as they are being continually rebuilt by two key cell types:

Osteoblasts – build new bone

Osteoclasts – destroy old bone

This is a great process. We all know of concrete buildings and indeed large metal structures which after a few years of standing start developing faults. This is exactly what would happen to our bones without an ongoing remodelling process.

The two types of cells are kept in very careful balance. Obviously in early life when the skeleton is growing the osteoblasts are winning and bones are getting longer and stronger.

Once growth stops there is still a balance in favour of building as more and more calcium is put into the bones making them stronger and stronger.

Peak strength is reached by 30 years of age and there is a very very slow decline from thereon.

In women after the menopause due to the fall in oestrogen levels this bone loss is accelerated. Bone is lost in most women at a rate of 1% of bone mass per year.

There are obviously loads of things which affect how quickly bone loss occurs:

Genetic – family history of osteoporosis is important

Drugs – some tablets e.g., steroids are damaging

Age of menopause – early menopause accelerates loss

Hormone Replacement Therapy – can be bone protective

Parathyroid hormone is one of the key hormones that controls the osteoblasts and osteoclasts. The mechanism of action is complicated.

Osteoblasts have a receptor on them which allows the PTH peptide to attach. The end result is the formation of more osteoclasts and therefore more resorption (destruction) of bone.

Osteoporosis is a massive problem particularly for the elderly as it increases the risk of fractures after falls particularly in the hip and wrist.

Spinal fractures can happen spontaneously causing severe back pain and are responsible for old people sometimes bending over – the so-called Dowager's hump.

It must be stressed that this effect of PTH on bone strength is really really slow.

However a few important facts are clear about the bones and parathyroid disease:

1. If you take patients who have been diagnosed with parathyroid disease and watch them for 10 years (without operating) then at the end of that time 50% will have developed osteoporosis

2. It is not possible to predict who will develop osteoporosis as the risk of developing it is not related to either the calcium or PTH level at diagnosis

3. Women are at greater risk of developing osteoporosis with parathyroid disease than men.

4. It is possible to develop osteoporosis at a very young age – even in the 40s – with parathyroid disease if it is not recognised and treated.

5. A bone density scan is a useful baseline study – particularly if patients have other risk factors or the diagnosis has been delayed.

6. Bone strengthening medicines e.g., bisphosphonates (Alendronic Acid etc) do NOT prevent patients with osteoporosis from getting worse if they also have parathyroid disease. This is common sense really – nature is stronger than a little tablet.

Bone pain – a common symptom with parathyroid disease is not thought to be directly due to the osteoporosis element even though some writers have tried to suggest it is.

The key feature of bone pain in parathyroid disease is that patients usually describe it as being pretty constant and in the middle of bones – particularly the long bones like the humerus and femur (arm and thigh bones). Arthritis pains are more likely to be felt in the joints themselves.

The good news is that as the bone pain is NOT due to the osteoporosis it vanishes as soon as the parathyroid tumour is removed.

I have seen some really dramatic cases – one lady in her mid 50s came having been on morphine for her bone pain for several years. She had been mis-diagnosed by a rheumatology doctor as having arthritis.

Fortunately for her a new rheumatology consultant noticed a slightly elevated calcium and suggested the correct diagnosis.

At this stage she had been off work with the bone pain for nearly 2 years and was taking large quantities of painkillers including the morphine – none of which were really working.

I operated on her removing a 3cm parathyroid tumour. The following morning she woke up and realised she was completely pain free. All her bone pain had vanished – and never came back.

She almost ran out of the hospital a new and rejuvenated woman leaving behind the morphine.

Parathyroid Glands and Vitamin D

This is a hugely complicated area and there are many different views.

I will try and provide a guide as to the key facts and also highlight areas where there is controversy.

Vitamin D is essential in the human body. Like all vitamins we cannot actually make them – this is the very definition of vitamin – a substance vital for life.

There are two sources of vitamin D – sunlight shining on the skin and from the diet.

Once we have vitamin D in the body it helps the intestine absorb calcium from the diet. Low vitamin D means that the gut will struggle to absorb calcium from food. Increasing vitamin D will generally mean that more calcium is absorbed from the diet.

Long term deficiency of vitamin D is not good for the health of the bones. In children the bones become soft and can bend – a condition called rickets. In adults the bones thin and become fragile – osteomalacia.

Vitamin D has become easier to measure in recent years although it is quite an expensive test for laboratories to undertake. We have increasingly seen patients with parathyroid disease and also in the general population with low vitamin D levels.

If you are healthy but have low vitamin D levels it is a good idea to boost them up by either getting more sunshine or taking vitamin D supplements.

Patients with primary parathyroid disease have high calcium levels and often have low vitamin D levels. There is a theory that the low vitamin D is part of the body's defence mechanism for the disease – by lowering vitamin D the absorption of calcium from food is reduced thereby reducing the calcium level.

I am not convinced by this theory as it ignores the facts that firstly the parathyroid glands are really rather good at their thermostat job and secondly that the body contains a vast calcium store in the bones where excess PTH can easily get some more calcium from if the intestine doesn't absorb as much.

The question I am often asked is whether patients should have low vitamin D levels corrected prior to having surgery. Here I have always been quite cautious and recommended waiting till after surgery.

However, there is emerging evidence that correcting vitamin D levels is absolutely safe to do. Obviously there may be some patients where this will increase the calcium level slightly but if symptoms worsen or calcium levels go up further the vitamin D can always be stopped.

Certainly after successful parathyroid surgery replacing vitamin D is a good idea to help towards rebuilding the bones.

www.ingramcontent.com/pod-product-compliance
Lightning Source LLC
Chambersburg PA
CBHW070719180526
45167CB00004B/1539